AF326980

about joe r:

I'm taking full responsibility for discovering joe r. He's a poet's poet— he tells the truth whether you want to hear it or not. joe truly cares and it shows in his writing— he cares about his art, he cares about his friends, and he cares about the world around him. joe's first chapbook, *gay in the head,* shows his philosophical side; his second chap, *i'm bettrr now,* shows his versatility; and his (ultimate) book, *the jeff book,* shows his honesty and insight. joe just gets better and better. He writes with conviction— he hates the injustices and he hates the suffering he sees going on around him. joe r is a class act, a good guy to have on your side, and, man, can he write! I should know, I discovered him.

— DAVE CHRISTY, *ALPHA BEAT PRESS*

joe's unique style will take you to the core of the matter...

— ANA CHRISTY, QUEEN OF THE UNDERGROUND

In an era of academic poetasters, devoid of blood & fire, & post-beat imitators w/their tributes & inadvertent send-ups of dead hipsters, joe r is a vibrant, incandescent voice, owing little to tradition or literary convention.

— ROBERT L. PENICK, *CHANCE MAGAZINE*

joe r is one of the most original and insightful poets writing today. His work never fails to make me think, make me laugh, or break my heart.

— DANIEL CROCKER, AUTHOR OF *PEOPLE EVERYDAY*

also by joe r:

r.l. nichols & faggot friends & poesy pals [1994]
(with R.L. Nichols, Michael Hathaway, Kevin Hibshman and L.E. Ward)
th'addvenchurzza scab boy [1994]
metaphors [1994]
(with bobby star and jim d)
gay in the head [1995]
White Boy Comes 2 Rumble: Gets Creamed By Gayboy [1995]
(with Paul Weinman)
Henry [1995]
(with Nathan Beaty)
Afrika [1995]
i'm bettrr now [1996]
when i waz parta the strayt wurld [1996]
posey [1996]
THE JEFF BOOK [1996]
Start a Fire or Die [1997]
1 night in the box [1997]
Smoke [1997]
allwayz judge a book by its covrr [1998]

do
yu
know.
what
distortion.
sowndz
like.

an urban legend

joe r

Green Bean Press
New York
1998

For information contact:
Green Bean Press, P.O. Box 237, New York, NY 10013
(718) 302-1955 phone/fax
gbpress@earthlink.net

isbn 1-891408-07-0

First Printing

Photo of the author by Ana Christy, 8/16/98
Design by Ian Griffin

The author would like to thank Keith Rosson
for the title of this book.

for
David
and
Ian—
in
a
world
of
punks
and
ass
holes,
2
fellow
travelers
worth
their
salt.

If on the journey of life a man can find a wise and intelligent friend who is good and self-controlled, let him go with that traveler; and in joy and recollection let them overcome the dangers of the journey.

—The Dhammapada, 328

corey'd
pisss
'er
pants.
jus'
ta
fukk
w/theyr
mindz.
they
came
arownd
at
7AM.
she
wantd
ta
pisss
at
6:45.
whattsa
matta?
yu
can'
holdit
fur a
louzy
stinkin'
15 minitts--
they'd
curss.
no--
she
thot.
n'd skweeeee
eeeeez
as hard

as she
culd.
like
maxwell
howss coffee
she waz
goooood.
ta
the
last
dropp.

corey
wazn't
a
ree
tard.
she
jus'
aktd
like
1.

i'll
bett.
yu
waz
a
beauty.
in
yur
day--
that 1
attendant
maria
wuld
say.
folks
uze
ta say.

corey
lookt
like
that
actress.
ruby
dee.
a reeeeee
eeeeal
hed
turnrr.
onna
satrrday
nite.
corey
jus'
lookt
like
corey
now.
7
dayz.
a
week.
n hedz
jus'
turnd.
rite
passt
'er.

corey
didn't
mind.
her
roomate.
priscilla.
eevn tho.
her
mind
had

deteriorated.
ta sumthin'.
akin.
ta a
skwash.
evry
time
wunnathoze
yung girlz'd
cum in.
ta change
the
sheets.
urrr empty
a bed
pan.
evry othrr
wurd.
outta
priscilla's
mowth.
waz
fukk.
urrr asss.
urrr sperm
bank.
corey
luuuuuuvd.
fukk n
asss
talk.
it ment
stubburn.
it ment
life.
yu go
girl--
corey
thot.
especially
w/sooooo
much

deth.
in the
room.

nursin'
home.
corey
thot
that
waz
funny.
the use
a the
wurd
home.
fur this
place.
nuthin'
like
the
homez
she
remembrrd.
w/kidz.
n noize.
n goooooo
oooood
food
smellz
waftin'.
the
food
heyr
smelld
like
#2.
the
#2
she
made
aftrr

her kidz
calld.
evry
othrr
week.
iff they
remembrrd.
corey
alwayz
remembrrd.
theyr waz
nuthin'
elss
ta do.
butt
remembrr.
we luv yu
momma--
they'd
say.

corey
had
2
kidz.
the
last
time
she
lookt.
a
boy
n a
girl.
samuel.
aftrr
'iz
fathrr.
n elisha.
aftrr
god-knowz

-what-the-
hell.
the 1 thing.
corey culdn't
remembrr.
fine
tuning's
a
thing.
a
the
past--
she
thot.

samuel
waz
alott
like
hiz
fathrr.
a
good
hardwurkin'
man.
w/the
personality.
of a
lettuss.
he had
a
wife.
n littl
boy.
who
were
also
vegetablz.
samuel
sold
thoze

thingz.
yu
hang
in
yur
car.
ta make
it
smelll.
good.
they
made
corey
choke.
butt
what'd
she
know.

elisha
didn't
hav
much
lukk.
w/men.
like
'er
prezent
boy
frend.
leonard.
he
waz
a
decent
enufff
guy.
like
he
didn't
beat

elisha
urrr
nuthin'.
he
jus'
felt.
what's
hiz.
is
hiz.
what's
herz.
is
hiz.
what's
evry
buddy
elssz.
is
hiz.
'specially
wallets.
n
purssz.
n
unlokkt
carz.
n
stufff.

he
seemz
allergik.
ta
wurk--
corey
sed.
once.
concernin'
leonard.
he's

oil.
n the
wurk's
watrr.
sumthin'
don't
smelll
rite--
she
went
on.
'bowt
a man.
afrayd.
of a
littl
dirt.
n
ree
sponsi
bility.
butt
leonard
didn't
much
kayr.
fur
dirt.
urrr
corey's
thots.
he
waz.
a
lion.
urrr at
leeeeeast.
he
thot
so.

corey'd
sit.
in
the
showrr.
w/'er
floppy
boobiez.
n
saggy
butt.
n
try
nott
ta
think.
abowt
how
the
wurld.
takes
evrything.
eventually.
'cept
yur
pride.
n i
baaaaaa
aarely
gott
hold
a
that--
she thot.
as a
20 yr old
girl.
washt
'er
privats.
w/a
ragg.

dammm
that
hurts--
corey'd
yell.
bett she
don't
rubb.
her
own
hoochie.
that
hard--
she
thot.

the
attendants
didn't
like
the
old
folks.
n the
old
folks
didn't
giv a
dammm
abowt
the
attendants.
eethrr.
they
were
yung.
n naive.
n vibrant.
n afrayd
the
deth

stink
mite
cum offf.
corey'd
shit
'er pants.
on
purpuss.
jus' so
they'd
hav.
a littl
bit a
her.
undrrneeth
theyr
fingrr
nailz.
ta take
home.
ta theyr
wivez.
n huzbandz.
n kidz.

corey
didn't
like
nuthin'.
urrr
nooooo
buddy.
at the
home.
the
stafff
waz
mostly.
yung
white.
trash

girlz.
who
smelld.
like
baby
powdrr.
n the
previuss
nite's
sex.
sumhow.
they
thot.
they
were
abuv it
alll.
YU
wipe.
MY
asss--
corey'd
think.
when she
spied
them
smiiiiilin'.

1
day.
this
kid
started
cummin'
arownd.
who's
the
boy--
corey
askt.
oh.

sum
lozer
ree
tard.
frum
the
hi
skool.
we
gotta
giv
a
jobb
ta--
maria
replied.
hiz
name's
billy.

corey
jus'
gave
maria.
wunna
her
looks.
like
ya
culd
diffrr
entiate.
1
lozer
reetard.
frum
anuthrr.
in
this
place.
corey'd

putt
her
munny
(iff
she
had
any).
on
the
new
blood.

n
billy
wazn't
a
ree
tard.
he
waz
17.

billy
waz
in
wunna
thoze
skool-
wurk
programz.
he'd
cum
ta
the
home.
evry
day.
alittl
aftrr
1PM.

ta sweep
the
floorz.
n
stufff.
he
lissnd
ta
muzik.
w/'iz
tape
playrr.
n hed
fonez.
beee
boppin'
arownd--
corey'd
say.
while he
wurkt.
watchin'
him.
waz the
1
thing.
in this
hole.
that
made
her
smile.

billy
worr
rippt
upp
crappy
jeanz.
n
'iz

tennrrz
was
fulla
holez.
thinkin'
of
her
own
spoyld
rottnn
grand
babiez
corey
thot--
poor
chil'.

what
corey
didn't
know.
waz
that
billy
waz
a
punk.
he
had
nuthin'.
ta
hide.
crap
waz
hiz
anthem.
bettrr
ta
wear
yur
bruizez.

than
bury
'em--
he'd
say
latrr.

he
waz
diffrint.
frum
most
othrr
kidz.
corey
knew.
he
carried.
hiz
own
clowdz.

billy's
hair
stukk
strayt
upp.
like
a
porky
pine--
corey
thot.
the
1st
thing.
she
evrr
sed.
ta

him.
waz--
chil'.
yu look.
like a
porky
pine.
what's a
porky
pine--
billy
askt.
a ratt.
w/needlz.
'stedda
hair.
kool--
billy
smiled.
n
walkt
away.

billy
made
hiz
own
t
shirts.
he'd
paynt
wurdz
on
'em.
like
"kill
me".
"corporate
meat".
n
corey's

favorit--
"maggot
pod".
this
kid's
fukkt
upp--
she
thot.
corey
liked
fukkt
upp.

yaknow
chil'.
yu'r
fukkt
upp--
corey
sed.
ta
billy.
1
day.
kool--
he
smiled.
aggin.
then
walkt
away.
aggin.
this
kid's
1
tufff
egg--
she
thot.

corey
didn't
know
nuthin'.
'bowt
billy's
famly.
like
iff
he
had
a
momma.
urrr
nott.
butt
1
day.
she
decided.
he's
gonna
gett
1.
heyr.
taday.
now.
like
it
urrr
nott.

tufff
egg
urrr
nott.
corey
waz
intent.
on
crakkin'.

billy's
shell.
he
bekame
her
mission.
she
didn't
know.
urrr
kayr
much.
y.
she
jus'
needed.
ta
do.
ta
be.
fur
sumone.
helll
she
jus'
needed.

1
friday.
billy
waz
sweepin'.
in
corey's
room.
she
knew.
she
hadta
say.
sumthin'.

hey
chil'--
she
finally
sed.
i
gott
an
idea.
fur
wunna
them
t
shirts.
howz
'bowt
"lateral
hell".

billy
stoppt.
n
lookt
upp.
good--
corey
thot.
butt
now
what
the
hell.
am
i
gonna
say.

what's
it
meeean--

billy
askt.
ooohhhhh
i dunno--
corey
replied.
guesss
i thot.
it
jus'
sownded
gooooooood.
billy
shook.
'iz
hed.
SOWNDZZZ
gooood--
he
sed.
ya
don't
say.
shit.
like
that.
w/o
it
meeeanin'.
sumthin'.
urrr
yu'r
as
fukkt
upp
as
i
am.

lissn
heyr--

corey
yelld.
linez'd
been
crosst.
festrring
woundz.
rippt
open.

she
gott
pisst.
1st a
all--
corey
sed.
i'm an
old
woman.
who's
owt
livd.
evry
one.
n evry
thing.
inkludin'
'er
useful
nesss.
hell.
i
gott
drawzzz.
that
culd
be.
yur
grand
daddy--

she
emfasized.
pointing.
a narrr
rrld
arthritik
fingrr.

billy
jus'
turnd.
hiz
hed.
n
did.
that
walk
awaaay
thing.
aggin.
DAMM
YU--
corey
showtd.
as
he
diss
appeerd.
down.
the
halll.

as
time
passt.
billy
stilll
kep'
cummin'.
arownd.

in
spite
a
theyr
littl
diss
agreee
ment.
n
corey
wuldn't
say.
nuthin'.
abowt
that
day.
like
it
nevrr
happnnd.

it
wazn't
wurth
lozing.
a
frend.

1
day
while
sittin'.
owt.
in
the
halll.
corey
notisst.
how
rezidents'

luvd
onez'd
cum
vizit.
n
park
themselvz.
nex'.
ta
the
shadowz.

once.
the
shadowz'd
been
sum
thin'.
momma.
poppa.
brothrr.
sistrr.
bee
luvd
aunt.
corey
notisst.
how
the
luvd
onez'd
keep
on
talkin'.
like
nuthin'.
waz
the
mattrr.
like
the

shadowz.
waz
morrr.
than
shadowz.

the
shadowz.
wazn't
all
wayz.
shadowz.
that's
what
happnnz--
corey
thot.
when
yu'r
oldrr.
than
dirrt.
that's
what
happnnz.
when
ya
owt
liv
godd.

the
best
part.
a this
shit
hole.
fur
corey
at

leeeeast.
waz
the
patio.
wheyr in
the spring
n
summrr
time.
she
culd
sit
owt.
fur
evrrrr.
w/the
treez.
n
pree
tend
life.
'stedda
furgettin'
abowt
it.

1
day.
they
cutt
down.
3
a
corey's
treez.
fur
the
helluvit
i
guess--
she

told
billy.
corey
jus'
stayrd.
at
the
stumps.
misss
sing
lunch
n
dinnrr.
thoze
treez
wuld
nott
eat.
taday.
neethrr
wuld
she.

peeplz
iz
fukkt
upp--
corey
told
billy.
1
day.
mos'
think.
ya
die.
all at
1
time.
uh-uh--
she

shook
'er hed.
it's
alittl
bitt.
evry
day.
iff
yu'r
lukky.
the
body.
goez
1st.

if
yu'r
nott--
she
went
on.
yu
beekum.
wunna
theez.
n
w/a
grand.
sweeping
gesture.
of
her
arm.
corey
indicatd.
her
wurld.
the
denizenz.
of
shadow.

yaknow
chil'--
she
went
on.
i pray.
yu
nevrr
see
the
day.
when
all
yu
know
iz
hate.
n
disgust.
when
noooo
buddy
antici
pates.
yur
prezenss.
w/glee.
when
yur
own
babiez'd
just
as
soooooon
putt
ya.
on the
mantl.
w/ded
flowrrz.

yu'd
bettrr
go.
chil'.
ya
dunn
gonn.
n
made.
an
old
lady.
spowt.
alotta
foooooo
oolish
nesss.
taday--
corey
chukkld.
t'her
selff.
as
she
realized.
she'd
shit.
'er
pants
oh
boyhee
hee
hee.
i'm
hee.
lukkyheeee
eeeeehee
heehee-
she
almost
fell
outta

her
chayr.

then.
THEY
SAY.
i'm
lukky.
ta
be
aliiiiiive.
shiyyyyyy
yyyyt.
i'm
lukky
allrite.
i can't
eevn
take
a shit.
that's
solid.
n brown.
i ain't
gott
no
goddamm
cuntrol.
ovrr
my own
bodily
funktionz.
evry
buddy.
n
theyr
goddamm
sistrr.
stikks
theyr
goddfursaknn

handz.
in my
goddamm
bizzness.
like
it waz.
theyr own.
LUKKY.
ooooohhhhh
i'm
lukky--
n corey
lookt.
at the
floor.
quiet.
like it
waz
beautiful.
fur
once.

yu
go
gett
maria.
hunny.
tell 'er
corey's
lukk's
been
alittl
looooss.
taday--
corey
sed.
fukk
'er--
she
thot.
maria'd

been.
in tooo
oooo
good
a mood.
this
morning.
she
needed
flattnning.

on 'iz
way.
owt
the
door.
billy
remarkt--
now
i know.
whatcha
mean.
know
what
what
meanz--
corey
askt.
yu know--
billy
sed.
he
smiled.

a
few
dayz
latrr.
corey
ree

turnd.
frum
the
rec
room.
n theyr
it
waz.
on
'er
bed.
a
t
shirt.
w/bigg
jaggedy
lettrrz.
paintd.
on
it.
"lateral
hell".
it
sang.
she
smiled.

it
seemd
as
tho.
corey'd
passt.
sum
kinda
test.
w/billy
he'd
stopp
by.
evry

day.
ta
talk.
n
lissn.
that's
what
impresst
corey.
the
most.
abowt
billy.
he
lissnd.
reeeeee
eeeally
lissnd.
ta
whatcha
had.
ta
say.

it
pissst
corey
offf.
how
mos'
folks'd
smiiiiile.
n
shake
theyr
hedz.
n akt.
like they
waz
lissnin'.
ah-ha--

they'd
say.
urrr--
oh
yeeeeaaah.
once
inna
while.
she'd
slipp
stufff
in.
like
dikkweed.
n
douche
bagg.
jus' ta
see.
butt it
didn't
mattrr.
they
waz all
reddy
home.
infronna
the
tv.
see ya--
they'd
say.
on
the
way
owt.
fukk yu--
corey'd
think.

THIS.
waz
corey's
home.
THIS.
waz
corey's
tv.
the
only
way
owt.
waz
ded.

billy
didn't
say
stufff.

urrr
shake
'iz
hed.

urrr
smile.

he
jus'
lookt.
at
ya.
he
waz.
wheyr
yu
waz.

n
hiz
talk.
waz
diffrint.
tooo.
it
waz
morr.
than
jus'
mowth.
n
wurdz.
it
waz
morr.
than
jus'
billy.
it
waz
sumthin'.
abowt
the
way.
he
made
ya
think.
n
feeeeeeel--
corey'd
say
latrr.

it
waz
billy's
wurld.
versus.

kaka
wurld.

n
the
kaka
wurld.
didn't
inn
klude
momz.

billy
told
corey.
abowt
'iz
mom.
how
they'd
been
alone.
fur
yearz.
how
billy
nevrr
knew.
hiz
reeeee
eeeal
dad.
how
he
felt.
like
an
un
ansrrd
kwestion.

urrr
a
story.
w/o
a
climax.
i
neeeed.
a
climax--
billy
sed.
i
must
create
1.

billy's
mom.
waz
a
gooood
woman.
she'd
allwayz
been
theyr.
n all
wayz
luvd
him.
wunna
hiz
errliest
memriez.
waz
her.
holdin'
him.
inna
rokkin'

chayr.
singin'--
men on
the
flying
trapeze.
"he
flotes
thru
the
ayr.
w/the
greatest
of eeeez"--
momz'd
sing.
"that
darin'
yung man.
on the
flappin'
trypeez."

momz'd
fukk
it
upp.
on
purpuss.
she
waz
funny.
that
way.
they'd
both
laff.
n laff.
til
it
hurt.

n
it
all
wayz
hurt.
eventually.
eevn
as
a
kid.
billy
lernd.
theyr's
sum
thin'.
bee
hind.
evry
smiiile.
sum
thin'
badd.
urrr
as
billy's
stepp
dad
calld
it--
reality.
butch
had no
time.
fur
fooooo
oolish
nesss.
billy
had no
time.
fur
butch.

evrything
turnz.
ta
shit--
billy
thot.

butch
wazn't
a
badd
guy.
urrr
a
good
guy.
he
waz
just.
a
guy.
momz
happnnd.
ta
luv.

he's
a
diffrint
boy--
momz'd
say.
ta
butch.
when
he'd
bitch.
abowt
billy's
hayr.

urrr
the
muzik.
he
lissnd
ta.
urrr
the
way
he'd
jus'
sitt
n
staaaaayr.

butch
didn't
hav.
much
use.
fur
diffrint
boyz.
he
didn't
hav.
much
use.
fur
boyz.
period.
jus'
beeeeer.
n
carz.
n
motrr
cyklz.
butch'd
giv
billy.

a
hard
time.
abowt
bein'
17.
n nott
havin'.
hiz
licenss.
wheelz.
is
freedum.
n
freedum.
is
a man's
prrre
eee
rogativ.
urrr
sumthin'
like
'at--
butch'd
say.

butch'd
nevrr
leav
billy.
alone.
he
waz
allwayz
eggin'
'im
on.
like
he
wantd.

-050-

ta
fite.
that's
all
butch
culd
undrr
stand.
waz
fite.
n
yell.
lowwwwd.
n
be
obnoxiuss.
n
stufff.

billy
nevrr
fawt.
he'd
jus'
sitt
theyr.
kwiet.
n
take
it.
faggott--
butch'd
yell.
assshole--
billy
thot.

this
scenario.
played

ittself
owt.
hundreds
a
timez.
once.
jus'
ta be
a
shit.
billy
blew
butch.
a
kiss.
neeeeeed
lesss
ta
say.
the
intellektual
giant.
butch
waz.
culdn't
grasp.
the
humor.
a
the
situation.

butch
grabbd
billy.
by
the
shirt.
n
slammd
'im.

agginst
the
wall.
billy
jus'
smiled.
n gave
butch
wunna
hiz.
what
momz
calld--
cold
steeeeel
looks.

butch
lett
billy
go.
down
deeep.
he
waz.
a
wuss.
wunna
theez
dayz--
he
grumbld.
yeah--
billy
thot.
wunna
theez
dayz.

no
buddy
knew.
what
waz
bee
yond.
the
cold
steeeeel
look.
no
buddy.
wantd
ta.

ya
don't
haffta.
be
old.
ta
be
ded--
billy
sed.
1
day.
it
helps--
corey
ree
plied.

kinda
weeeeird--
billy
went
on.
jus'

when.
ya
gett.
the
hang.
a
this
livin'
thing.
it's
time.
ta
go.
AAAAmen--
corey
sed.
just
as
priscilla.
reecht
down.
inta
her
diaprr.
fur
sum
poop.

she
wulda.
ate
it.
tooo.
iff
billy
hadn't
cawt
'er.
in
time.

n
then.
1
day.
billy
kwit
cummin'.
maria
sed.
she
herd.
he'd
runn.
away.
frum
home.
butch
the
bastrrd--
corey
thot.
trash--
maria
sed.
refrrin'
ta
billy.
i
knew.
he
waz.
a
lozer.
n a
ree
tard.
frum
the
gett-go.

this
waz.
a
very
delikat
matrr.
fur
corey.
how
do.
ya
tell.
the
person.
who
wipes.
yur
asss.
onna
daily
basis.
ta
fukk
offf.
fukk
offf
maria--
corey
sed.
billy
wulda
been
prowd.

corey
laid.
wide
awake.
in
bed.
all

nite.
unabl
ta
sleeep.
thinkin'
abowt
billy.
wheyr
he
waz.
what
he
waz
doin'.
how
many
timez.
he'd
wisht.
he
waz
ded.

that
is.
until
she
herd.
alittl
tap
tap
tap.
on
the
window.
it
waz
billy.

what
the
hell
yu
doin'.
wheyr
the
hell
yu
been.
who
the
hell
yu
hangin'
arownd
with--
corey
almost
skreeee
eeamd.
simmrr
down
ma--
billy
ansrrd.
it
waz.
hiz
next
line.
that
corey'd
nevrr
furgett--
yu
wanna
cum
w/me.

as
iff.
she
had.
a
choyss.
corey
culd
whiiii
iiile
away.
the
hourz.
enamord.
by that
asss
hole
maria's
prezenss.
urrr
face.
the
freedum.
of
nott
knowing.

the
home.
waz
a
safe
place.
safe
ta
sitt.
n
die.
corey'd
be
nutts.

ta
leav
all
that.

how
the
helll.
yu
gonna
gett
me.
outta
heyr.
i
can
baaaaaa
aayrly
walk--
corey
whined.
i
bett.
iff i
litt.
a
match.
undrr
yur
asss--
billy
sed.
yu'd
find.
a
way.
sooooo
pree
tend.
jus'
then.

they
herd.
maria
cummin'
down.
the
halll.
corey
culdn't.
a
flown.
owt
that
window.
any
fastrr.

the
lord
do
wurk.
in
mysteriuss
wayz.
don't
he
boy--
corey
chukkld.
butt
billy
didn't
hear.
he'd
gonn
on.
ahed.
walkin'.
he
waz
allwayz

leedin'.
the
way.
walkin'.
corey
hadd.
no
choyss.
but
ta
follow.
walkin'.

they
walkt.
fur
what
seemd.
like
milez.
ta
corey.

they
ended
upp.
in
a
crutty
sektion.
a
U
street.
lord
godd
all
mitey--
corey
sed.
what

happnnd.
ta
this
naybur
hood.
timez
change--
billy
answrrd.
peepl
don't.

ree
membrr--
billy
went
on.
yu
havn't.
been
owt.
a
that
home.
fur
yearz.
bakk
in
yur
day.
it
payd.
fur
folks.
ta
hide.
the
uggly.
now.
it
don't.

in
uthrr
wurdz--
corey
sed.
as
long
as.
theyr's
peepl.
content.
ta
eat
shit.
theyr'll
be
morrr
than
enufff.
willin'.
ta
shuvl
it.

that's
itt--
billy
smiled.
i
think.
yu'll
like
itt.
heyr.

shit.
as
long
as.
theyr

ain't.
nooooo
maria--
corey
thot.
i'd
liv.
in
haydeez.

billy
waz
livin'.
in
wunna
thoze
oooold
howzez.
corey
all
wayz
luvd.
as
a
kidd.
'cept
billy's
waz
missin'.
a
few
windowz.
a
brikk.
heyr
n
theyr.
n the
porch
wazn't
attacht.

tooo
goood.
we'r
gonna
fixx
it
upp--
billy
sed.
yu.
n
what
army--
corey
thot.

she
culd
imagin
snow.
blowin'
thru
holez.
in
the
roof.
her
arthritis.
startd
aktin'
upp.
she
clozed
'er
eyez.
n
prayd.
fur
divine
intrr
vention.

nuthin'
happnnd.

how
much.
they
jipp
yu.
fur
this
place.
evry
month--
corey
askt.
nuthin'--
billy
ansrrd.
rathrr
strayt
faced.
whatchu
mean
child--
corey
askt.
jus'
what
i
sed.
nuthin'.
we
don't
pay.
no
rent--
billy
ssssmiiii
iiiiled.

it's
a
skwat.
corey's
arthritis
kikkt.
inta
2nd
gear.

we'r
wunna
the
lukky
onez
tooo--
billy
went
on.
we
gott
runnin'
watrr.
elektricity.
a haff
wayz
deecent
hott
watrr
heatrr.
only
thing
is
(corey
knew
she
didn't
wanna
hear
this)
the

furnass.
don't
wurk.
so
good.
it
only
cumz
on.
when
it's
really
reeeally
reeeeeeally
cold.

3rd gear.

hitlrr.
shulda
hadd.
such
lukk--
corey
thot.

billy
brawt
corey.
inta
the
howss.
eevn
bee
forrr.
her
eyez.
hadd
time.

ta
fokus.
who'z
dee
oooold
niggrr
lady--
ree
verbrr
rrated.
akrosss
the
room.

i
ain't
stayin'.
in
da
saaaame
howss.
wit'
no
niggrrz--
meeka
continued.
n
i
don't
stay.
in the
same
howss.
w/asss
holezzz--
anuthrr.
morrr
delikate
voyss.
deeklayrd.
soooo it

looks
like.
we'r
eevn
steevn.
we all
stay.
settld.
then
IT.
the
delikat
thing.
walkt
ovrr.
ta
corey.

IT
walkt.
like
a
girl.
IT
talkt.
like
a
girl.
IT
eevn
muuuuuu
uuuuu
uuvd.
like
a
girl.
butt
IT
wazn't
no girl.
at

least.
in the
traditionl
senss.

deeeeeear
godd.
giv
me
strength--
corey
prayd.
giv
me.
the
powrr.
ta...
hiiii
hun--
IT
sed.
i'm
misss
tim.
wunnnnn
drrful
to
meet
yu.
pleaz
pardon
mr.
meeka.
he's
an
idiot
savant.
morrr
idiot.
than
savant.

butt
he's
gott.
a jobb.
n pretty
blue
eyez.
so
we
lett
him
stay.

misss
tim
winkt.
at
meeka.
who
then
pree
tended.
ta
vomitt.
what
lookt
like.
niagrra
fallz.
ha
ha.
funny
mr. meeka.
yu
know.
yu
want
it--
misss
tim
chukkld.

then
kisst
her
fingrr.
n
tucht.
a
rathrr
shapely
bee
hynd.

misss
tim.
pulld
corey
asiiide.
we
girrrlz.
hav
to
stikk
togethrr--
she
sed.
don't
wurry
hun.
he tried
pulling.
that
saaaaame
shit.
w/me.
he's
a
cuntrol
freak.
i
simply
kikkt.

hiz
bigottd
asss.
dowwwwn
thoze
stepps.
yu
see
heyr.
akrosss
the
street.
n arowwwwnd
the
cornrr--
misss
tim
winkt.
at
meeka.
aggin.
but
he
wazn't
lookin'.

now.
the
poooooor
dear.
can't
eevn
shit.
w/o
shakin'.
in
my
prezensss--
misss
tim
sed.

sooooo
yu
go
girrrl.
like
the
song
sez.
expressss
yur
selff.
misss
tim.
gottcha
covrrd.
misss
tim's
alll
ovrr
THAT
foool.
like
a
wett
wash
ragg.

maybe
so.
butt
meeka
didn't
hear.
he
waz
allreddy
heded.
fur
the
door.
he

didn't
kayr.
ta
be
arowwwnd.
nooooo
morrr.
at
leeeeeast.
until
misss
tim.
simmrrd
dowwwwww
wwwwn.
fony
bitch--
he
thot.
as
he
litt.
that
1st
cigrrett.
in
the
chilly.
nite.
air.

misss
tim.
chattd
on.
n
on.
n
on.
she
didn't

reeeeeeally
kayr.
iff
yu
lissnd.
urrr
nott.
corey
culd
telll.
misss
tim.
waz
as
much.
inta
cuntrol.
as
that
meeka
fella.
probly
morrr.
a
match.
made
in
heven--
corey
mumbld.
t'herselff.
as
she
thot.
abowt
othrr
thingz.

wantin'.
ta
cuntrol.

cumz
frum
hate--
corey
thot.
n
hate.
frum
feeeear
n
igg
noranss.
n
feeeear
n
igg
noranss.
frum
pain.

lookin'
arown'
the
rooom.
corey
saw.
lottsa
pain.

corey
knew
pain.

i.
can
liv.
w/that--
she
thot.

alluva
suddnn.
corey
realized.
miss
tim.
had
flittd.
away.
she'd
spied.
morr
willing
n
appropriat
targetts.

exkuze
me--
a
voysss
sed.
frum
outta.
the
fringez.
it
broke.
corey's
traaaain.
a
thot.
yu
must
be
corey.
name's
helen--
it
sed.
i'm

a
frend.
a
billy's.
he's
told
me.
aaallll
abowt
yu.
the
home.
maria.
priscilla.
how
yu
saved
hiz
life.
evrything--
she
went
on.
sum
nites.
i
didn't
think.
he'd
evrr
shuttupp.
n go.
ta
bedd.

n
yu
know
billy--
helen
sed.

anything.
morrr
than
3
wurdz.
is
an
eevent.
wo
wo
woooo--
corey
replied.
whatta
yu
talkin'
abowt.
me.
savin'
HIZ
life.

then
theyr
waz.
a
silenss.

helen
waz
beauuu
uuti
fulll.

bald.

butt
beauti
fulll.

like
a
saint.

she
bitt
her
lowrr
lipp.
kep'
lookin'
dowwwwwn.
at
'er
boots.
teeeearz
welld.
oh
shit--
she
sed.
i
fukkt
upp.
aggin.
i
allll
wayz.
fukk
upp.
jus'
calll
me.
fukk
upp.

helen
beekame.
bigg
blue

-084-

vulnrrabl
marbl
eyez.
she
broke
corey's
hart.

don't
yu
wurry.
chil'--
corey
sed.
as
she
took.
helen's
hand.
n
skweeeeeezd.
yur
seekret's
safe
w/me.
helll.
i'll
probly.
furgett
it.
5
minnitts
latrr.
anywayz.

helen
chukkld.
waaaaaay
tooo
much.

loooooong.
n
lowwwd.
it's
the
poizon.
cummin'
owt--
corey
thot.

this.
is
aaallll
abowt.
yu--
helen
managed
ta
say.
whattaya
mean
chil'--
corey
askt.
this
skwat.
the
peepl.
r littl
community--
helen
went
on.
nunn
of
uss'd
be
heyr.
iff
it

wazn't
fur
yu.
urrr
shuld
i
say.
billy's
vision.
of
yu.

'skuze
me.
dear--
corey
sed.
butt
this
ooooold
lady's
brayn.
don't
wurk.
sooo
gooooood.
anymorrr.
now
whatthehell.
yu
talkin'
abowt.
i'm
sorry--
helen
blusht.
as she
smiiiled.
her
tufff
chikk

look.
waz
a
veneeeer.
masking.
the
delikats.
inn
side.

that's
what.
i
ment.
when
i
sed.
yu
saved.
billy's
life--
helen
continued.
theyr
were.
a
cupla
timez.
w/butch
n
alll.
that
it
gott.
reeeeeeal
badd.
billy
had.
summa
hiz
mom's

valiumz.
alll
reddy.
ta
go.
butt
he
culdn't.
he
culdn't
leeeeav
yu.
he
sed.
he
culdn't
dissappoynt.
yu.

helen
told.
this
story.
like
it
waz
sumthin'.
she'd
thot
abowt.
fur
a
looooong
time.
n
didn't
like.
what
she
thot.

i
guesss.
i'm
jelluss--
helen
sed.
outta
the
blue.
seeee.
i
luv
billy.
hart
n
sooooole.

that's
goooood
chil'--
corey
interruptd.
billy
neeeeedz.
that.
he
neeeeedz
yu.
theyr's
nuthin'.
ta
be
jelluss
of.
no
no
nooooo--
helen
chukkld.
aggin.

yu
don't
gettit.
he
luvz
yu.
tooo.

helen
pauzed.
fur
a
moment--
billy
sez.
he
luvz
me.
like
a
girrrl
frend.
a
wife.
a
life
looooong
companion.
he
sez.
we'r
soooooole
mates.

butt
yu--
she
went
on.
he

can't
exx
playn.
he
duzzn't
undrr
stand.
the
attraktion.
allz
he
knowz.
is
that
yu.
must.
be
a
part.
of
hiz
life.
yu
MUST.
be
arownd.
he
can't
go
on.
a
singl
sekund.
with
owt.
yu.

THAT'S
what.
i'm
jelluss

of--
helen
sed.
as
she
lookt.
owt.
the
bay
window.
the
mystrry.
I
WANT.
TO
BE.
THE
MYSTRRY.
fur
chrissakes.
look
at
me.
bald.
n
tattood.
ruuuude.
i'v
dedikated
my
fukkin'
life.
ta
bein'
inn
exxplikabl.
n
unnknowwwwn.

now.
i

feeeel.
compart
mentliii
iiized.
pidgin
holed.
figgrrd
owt.
the
fukkin'
saaaaaaame.
as
evry
thing
elss--
helen
siiiiighd.
i
guesss.
i'm
just
anuthrr
kidd.
goin'
thru.
anuthrr
stage.
on
'er
way.
ta
bein'
anuthrr
wife.

ooohh.
i
wish.
i
hadd.
the

wizdum.
a
solomon.
dear--
corey
sed.
n
knewwww.
the
rite
thingz.
butt
i
don't.
i'm
jus'.
an
85
yr
old
woman.
who's
managed.
simply.
ta
wake
upp.
a
goooood
amownt.
a
dayz.

wish.
i
culd
make
it.
aaaalllll
bettrr--
corey

lookt.
inta
helen's
eyez.
allz
i
can
tell
ya.
is
don't
nevrr
furgett.
nuthin'.
ree
membrr.
n
lern.
n
theyr
ain't.
nuthin'
wrongg.
w/bein'.
anuthrr
wife.
as
long
as.
the
lethrr.
n
tattooz.
n
bald
hed.
r
theyr.
sumwheyr
undrr
neath.
the

apronz.
n
stringz.

n
ta
be.
kwite
honest.
w/ya--
corey
went
on.
yu
don't.
gott
shit.
figgrrd
owt.
pidgin
holed.
compart
mentlii
iiized.
dee
fined.
shiiiyyyt.
who
yu
think.
yu
r.
the lord
hizself.
chil'
theyr's
gonna
be
dayz.
when
ya

wish.
ya
culd
jus'
grabb.
a
handfulll.
n
hang
on.

christ--
corey
sed.
yu
ain't
eevn
20.
yett.
life'll
all
wayz.
be
a
mystrry.
to
ya.
chil'.
'specially
yur
own.
FLOTE--
corey
showtd.
that's
the
best
advice.
i
can

giv
ya.

flote.

iff
ya
can.

butt
i
don't
know.
iff
i
can--
helen
ree
plied.
neethrr
do
i--
corey
sed.
it's
aaallll
abowt
livin'
n
nott
knowin'.
it's
okay.
ta
be
afrayd.
shiiiyyyt
chil'--
corey
lafft.
i'm

afrayd.
evry
goddamm
day.
a
my
life.

then
how.
do
yu.
go
on--
helen
askt.
stoopidity--
corey
chukkld.
i'm
the
dummest
person.
i
know.
iff
alll.
thoze
suppozedly
grate
fee
losofrrz.
culdn't
figgrr.
it
owt.
then
how.
the
hell.

can
i.

i
wake
upp.
evry
mornin'.
keep
1
eye
clozed.
n
grope.
my
way.
thru.
the
darknesss--
corey
sed.
9 timez.
outta
10.
i
find
sumthin'.
that
10th
time.
i
don't.
i
jus'
gooooo
bakk.
ta
bedd.
probly
need
the

rest.
anywayz.
heeeee
heee--
they
both
lafft.
as
billy.
walkt
ovrr.

i
seee.
yu
2.
hav
mett--
he
sed.
i
told
helen.
yu
guyz'd
gett.
aloooong.
soooooo
what'v
ya
been
talkin'.
abowt.
thingz--
helen
answrrd.
yeah
thingz--
corey
chimed
inn.

well.
lett's
rapp
THINGZ
upp--
billy
sed.
corey.
yu'v
hadda
long
day.
n
neeeeed.
ta
gett.
ta
bedd.
NOW.

lissn
heyr.
ya
littl
pisss
ant--
corey
replied.
i
gott
drawz.
oldrr.
than
yu.
i'll
gooooo.
ta
bedd.
when
i
damm

well
pleeeeaz--
she
waz
smiiiiiilin'.
who
yu
think.
yu
r.
maria
the
2nd.

yeah--
billy
playd
alongg.
we'r
identikl
twinz.
alike.
in
evry
way.
'cept
her
dikk.
is
longrr.
than
mine.

corey
lafft.
soooooo
hard.
that.
she
haddta

lay.
on
the
cowch.
w/her
feet.
in
the
air.

n
it
waz
contagiuss.
pretty
soon.
evry
buddy.
in
the
room.
waz
laffin'.
at
corey
laffin'.

n
it
waz
good.

fur
once.

the
nex'
morning.
corey

waz
upp.
errrly.
she
nevrr
slep'.
welll.
in
straaaaange
placez.

that
meeka
fella
waz
upp.
tooo.
mornin'
mr.
meeka--
corey
sed.
fine
day.
may
as
welll
try.
n
be
hosspitabl--
she
thot.
asss
holez
hav.
a
mornin'.
tooo.

meeka
jus'
mumbld
sumthin'.
corey
culdn't.
undrr
stand.
n
porrrrd
sugrr.
in
hiz
cawfee.
maybe.
summa
that'll
seep.
inta.
hiz
disss
pozition--
corey
thot.

i
say.
goood
mornin'.
mr.
meeka--
corey
ree
peetd.
n
i
anssr.
goood
morning--
meeka
sed.

as
he
porrrrd.
n
stirrrd.
porrrrd.
n
stirrrd.

that
mus'
be.
sum
jobb.
yu
gott--
corey
sed.
tryin'
ta
make.
convrr
sation.
that
getts
ya
upp.
this
errly.
meeka
finally
stoppt
stirrrrin'.
n
glaaayyyyrr
rrrrd.
at
corey.

i
t'ink
my
affayrz.
is
MYYYY
bizznisss--
he
sed.
n
walkt
ovrr.
ta
the
tabl.
satt
down.
n
began
sipping.
hiz
cawfee.

the
way.
meeka
craydld.
hiz
cupp.
reeminded
corey.
of
a
littl
boy.
the
way.
her
littl
samuel.
uze

ta
cherrrr
rrish.
hott
coco.
on
coooold.
blustrry.
wintrr
morninz.

is
skoool
clozed
taday
momma--
sammy'd
ask.
exxcited.
on
the
verge.
a
bustin'.
outta
hiz
britchz.
corey
luuuuuuuvd.
when
she
culd
say.
yesssss.
YYYIIIPPPEEEE--
sammy'd
showt.
as
he
wirrrrld.
n

twirrrrld.
n
jumpt.
hiz
way.
arownd
the
kitchn.
hush
hush
chil'--
she'd
chide.
yur
poppa.
n
sistrr.
is
sleepin'.

corey
smiled.
thoze.
were
happy
timez--
she
thot.
lord
jeezus.
what'm
i
doin'--
she
siiiighd.
alowd.
do
yu
MIND--
meeka
sed.

i
gett
soooooo
few.
privat
moments.
in
dis
howsss--
he
went
on.
i
wuld
appreciate.
sum
kwiet.
iff
yu
feeeeel.
da
cumpulsion.
ta
speek.
wit'
yurselff.
pleeeeaz
do
so.
in
anuthrr
rooom.
T'ANK
yu.

corey
hadta
bite.
her
tung.

she
turnd.
ta
leav.
n
by
da
waaaay--
meeka
sed.
deyr's
dis
t'ing.
calld
a
lite
switch.
in
da
rest
rooom.
pleeeeeaz
uze
it--
meeka
smiled.
I
PAY.
d'elek
tricity.

corey
stoppt.
ded.

that
waz
it.

exkuse
me

sir--
corey
sed.
n
i
hope.
yu'll
pardnn.
an
ooooold
NIGGRR
lady.
fur
askin'.
butt
waz
yu
borrrn.
an
ASSS
hole.
urrr
is
it
sumthin'.
yu
lernt.
ovrr
a
period
a
tiiiime.

meeka
didn't
say
nuthin'.
fur
a
looooong
time.

he
lookt
down.
at
'iz
cawfee.
dis
is
abowt.
last
nite.
izn't
it--
he
sed.
it's
abowt.
alotta
nites--
corey
ree
plied.

i
drink.
a
lott.
TOOO
MUCH.
at
timez--
meeka
continued.
i
say
t'ingz.
dat
ain't
sooooo
true.
offf

da
poynt.
of
my
hed.

heeeee.
yu
meen
topp--
corey
chukkld.
that's
TOPP.
a
yur
hed.
hunny.
finally
sum
buddy.
who
manglz.
the
language.
as
much.
as
i
do.

n
iff
ya
lookt.
reeeeeeeal
hard.
ya
mite
a

sed.
meeka
smiiiled.

yu
ain't
frum.
this
cuntry.
r
yu--
corey
askt.
no--
meeka
ree
plied.
i
cum
frum.
da
soviet
union.
8
yrz
ago.
oooohhh
hhh--
corey
sed.
yu
wunna
them.
disso
dents.
no--
meeka
went
on.
i'm
aaahhhh.

what
yu
say.
homo
sekshul.

corey
lookt
confuzed--
sooooo
that's
y
yu.
n
him.
i
meen
her.
yaknow.
misss
jim.
urrr
kim.
urrr
whatevrr
the
helll.
its
name
is.
shit
NO--
meeka
ree
plied.
she
ain't
my
typ.

n
corey
lafft.
like
theyr
waz
no.
ta
morrow.

no--
meeka
sed.
aktually
billy's
my
typ.
dat's
how.
i
cum.
ta
liv.
heyr.
at
dis
flopp.
yu
meen
skwat--
cory
sed.
n
they
both
lafft.

heeee.
yu
know

sumthin'.
mr.
meeka--
corey
sed.
yu
ain't.
such
a
baaaaaaad
guy.
aftrralll.
butt
that
stilll.
don't
exkuse.
aaallll
that
niggrr
shit.
the
othrr
nite.
boooooooz.
has
a
way.
a
bein'.
a
truth
see
rummm.
iffya
know.
what
i
meen.

in
my
cuntry--
meeka
ree
plied.
peepl
t'ink.
ameriknn
blakks.
carry
gunnz.
do
dope.
make
karate.
n
danss.
pleeeeaz
akksept.
my
apologiez--
he
went
on.
butt
da
only
blakks.
i
knew.
as
a
child.
waz
in
moviez.
n
den
tv.
when
i

cum
heyr.
like
aaahhhh
shaff.
lemme
see.
dyno
miiiiiite.
mistrr
caw
TERRRRR.
aaahhhh
weeeezy.
yu
know.
yu
mus'
know
dem.

corey
didn't.
say
nuthin'.
meeka.
waz
rite.

he
waz
blond.

bluuuuue
eyed.

skiiinnny.

he
wazn't.

no
spy.

didn't
hav.
no
beeeeee
eard.

didn't
wayr.
no
biiigggg.
furry
hatt.

touché--
she
thot.

she
culd
telll.
by
the
look.
on
'iz
face.
that
meeka.
waz
seriuss.
he
thot.
she
aktually
knew.
theez
folks.
who

the
hell.
yu
talkin'
abowt--
she
askt.
i
don't
know.
nooooo
weeezy.
urrr
dyno
mite.
frum
adam.
tv
folks.
ain't
reeeeeal.
chil'.

butt
dey'r
blakk.
yu
shuld
know
dem--
meeka
ree
plied.
rathrr
confuuuzed.
do
yu
know.
evry
russian--
corey

askt.
evry
white
man.
womnn.
n
chil'.
n
as
far.
as
that
tv
shit's
consrrnd--
corey
waz
on.
a
rollllll.
that's
when
billy.
n
helen.
came
in
ta.
the
rooom.

i
thot.
yu
2'd
be
dukin'.
it
owt.
by
now--

billy
sed.
naaahhhh--
corey
ree
plied.
jus'
a
littl.
missssss
undrr
standin'.
n
anywayz--
she
went
on.
i'm
a
luvrr.
nott
a
fightrr.
jus'
as
soooooooon.
bulll
shit.
my
way.
outta.
the
situation.
than
take.
an
asssss
wuppin'.

rite
mr.

meeka--
corey
askt.
riiiite--
he
ree
plied.
aaallll
misss
undrr
standingz.
bool
shits.
ovrr
asss
woopingz.
any
tiiiiiime.

welll
welll
welll--
billy
sed.
so
yu
2'v
finlly
kisst.
n
made
upp.
that's
nice.
1
lesss
war.
ta
be
waged.
withinn

theez
walllz.
now.
iff
i
culd
jus'
gett
meeka.
ta
marry
tim.
we
mite
be.
ree
spektabl.

don't
hold.
yor
bresst--
meeka
ree
plied.
that's
breth.
mistrr
meeka--
corey
sed.
whatevrr--
he
smiiiiiled.
it
AIN'T
gonna
happnn.

welll--
billy
siiighd.
i
guesss.
we'r
aaallll
jus'
born.
ta
be.
white
trash.
then.

they
alll
lookt.
at
corey.
n
bustd
owt.
laffin'.

billy
excuuuzzd
himselff--
that's
honrrary.
in
yur
case.
m'am.

now
i
don't
meeeeen.
ta

telll.
yu
folks.
yur
bizznisss--
corey
sed.
w/a
strayt
face.
butt
ain't
yu
spoze.
ta
have.
a few
tirez.
on
the
frunt
porch.
n
a
cowch.
in
the
yard.
sum
rope.
sevrral
shott
gunnz.
a
nooss.
urrr
2.

helen
lafft.

soooooo
oooo
hard.
she
made.
thoze
littl
skweeky
noyzezzz.
like
when.
she
had.
asthma
attakks.
shitt.
wheyr's
my
inn
halrr--
she
gasspt.
as
she
ran.
outta
the
room.

congratulationz
folks--
billy
proklaymd.
yu'v
jus'
skored.
a
whopping
20%
lungg
capacity.

on
the
helen
moore
lafff
machine.
shutt
the
fukk
upp.
billy--
helen
sed.
stilll
giggling.
yu
killl
me.
i
know--
he
ree
plied.

okay.
whatevrr.
ANYwaaayzzz--
billy
stumbld.
aaallll
ovrr
the
place.
when
he
gott
flustrrd.
keep
a
looksee.
owt.

fur
the
copps--
he
sed.
i'm
surre.
between
corey's
famly.
n
my
stepp
fathrr.
they'r
owt.
in
fulll
forss.
probly
casin'
the
joynt.
as
we
speek.

jus'
ta
be
safe--
billy
went
on.
uze
the
bakk
door.
hopp
the
fenss.

n
gett
on
12th
streeet.
that
awta
throw
'em.
fur
awhiiiiiile.

reemembrr
the
lite
bizniss--
helen
chimed
in.
o
YEAH--
billy
sed.
don't
turn
on.
any
lites.
play
radioz.
singg.
danss.
NUTHIN'.
till
this
thingg.
blowz
ovrr.
we
gotta
make

'em
think.
nobuddy
livz
heyr.

n
corey--
billy
went
on.
yu
bettrr.
stay
putt.
heyr.
walkin'
iz
1
thingg.
butt
jumpin'
fensszzz.
iz anuthrr.
yeah
yeah
yeeeaaahhh--
she
ree
plied.
n
i
won't.
be
dancin'.
no
jiggz.
neethrr.

corey
felt.
like
she
waz
bein'
talkt
down
tooo.
aggin.
sorta
like
maria.
fightin'
'er
way.
bakk
in.

okay.
lett's
go--
billy
allwayz.
chekkt
'iz
pokketts.
beeforr
he
went.
any
wheyr.
nervuss
habbitt.
morr
than
any
thingg.
reemind
me.
ta

gett.
sum
smokes--
he
sed.
ta
helen.
i'm
allmost.
owt.

hey
mistrr
meeka--
corey
sed.
as
he
waz
abowt.
ta
walk
owt.
the
dooor.
yu
evrr.
been
ta
spain.

sumwhat
surprized.
by
the
kwestion.
meeka
ansrrd--
y
yesss.

3
timez.
madrid.
barcelona.
pamplona.
to
be
exxakt.

corey
putt
'er
hed
bakk.
clozed
'er
eyez.
n
smiiiiiled.
pleeeaz
telll
me.
it
waz
beauuuuti
fulll--
she
sed.
eevn
iff.
ya
haffta
lie.
pleeeeeeeaz
telll.
me.
it
waz
beauuuutifulll.

it
is
beauti
fulll--
meeka
sed.

thank
ya--
she
ree
plied.

y
do
yu
ask--
meeka
wundrrd.
oooohhhhh
i
saw.
this
tv
show.
once--
corey
reeplied.
abowt
spain.
n
madrid.
n
thoze
plazaz
they
gott.
folks
waz
walkin'.

n
talkin'.
n
havin'.
a
grand
oooole
time.
drinkin'.
them
littl
cupps.
a
cawfee.

the
memry.
a
that
show.
n
the
place.
n
thoze
folks.
n
that
goddammmd
cawfee.
kep'
me
aliiive.
fur
yeeeearz--
she
pawzd.
i
jus'
haffta
beeleev.

it's
reeeeeeeally.
that
beauuutifulll.

sum
thinggz.
shuld
simply
allwayzzz.
be
beauuuuti
fulll--
corey
continued.
as
she
thot.
abowt
herselff.
the
home.
n
what
waz
lefft.
of
her
life.

butt
theyr's
hope--
meeka
sed.
almost
as
iff.
he
culd

reed.
her
mind.

hope--
corey
thot.
what
a
funny.
littl.
wurd.
sumthin'
i
havn't
herd.

urrr
seeen.

urrr
sed.

urrr
felt.

fur
yeerz.

billy
waz
walkin'.
down
the
street.
when
alluva
suddn.
he
herd--

hey
man.
yu
gotta
smoke.
billy
lookt
down.
it
waz.
a
stikk
man.

kidz.
all
ovrr.
the
wurld.
draw.
stikk
peepl--
billy
thot.
this
is.
a
liiiiiive
1.

at
leeeeast.
he
appeard.
ta
be.

yu
contem
playtin'.

the
ree
lidguss
ramifi
kationz.
a
givin'
me.
a
smoke--
the
stikk
man
asktd.
urrr
r
ya
just
enamrrd.
by
my
beauuuuu
uuuty.

sorry--
billy
sed.
n
handed.
the
stikk
man.
a
smoke.
he
tried.
ta
lite
it.
himselff.
butt

waz
shakin'.
tooo
much.
SHIT--
he
yelld.
billy
litt
it.
fur
'im.
iff
yu'r
wundrrin'--
the
stikk
man
went
on.
this
ain't.
the
latest
jane
fonda
diet.
it's
AIDS.
feeeeeeel
free.
ta
staaare.
a
hole.
thru
my
face.

sorry--
billy

ree
peetd.
that's
okay.
man.
i
gett
it.
alll
the
time--
the
stikk
man
sed.
at
leeeeast.
yu
didn't
spitt.
on
me.

n
by
the
way--
the
stikk
man
lookt.
puzzld.
do
yu
know.
what
distortion.
sowndz
like.

huh--
billy
sed.

i
guesss.
it's
my
turn.
ta
be
sorry--
the
stikk
man
chukkld.
it's
jus'.
that
i
managed.
ta
sleeeeep.
a
few
hourz.
last
weeeek.
n
i
hadd.
this
dreeeeam.

the
stikk
man.
took
a
draaaaa

aaagg.
on
hiz
cigrrett.

then
cawfft.
abowt
52
timez.

he
waz
crowcht
down.
agginst
a
walll.
billy
had.
ta
crowch
down.
nex'
ta
him.
he
didn't.
wanna
misss.
a
wurd.

like
i
waz
sayin'--
the
stikk
man

mumbld.
bee
forr
i
waz
sooooo
ruuuuudely
intrr
ruptd.
by
what's
lefft.
a
my
lungz.
i
had.
this
dreeeam.
n
theyr
waz.
a
lady.
in
it.
n she
askt--
do
yu
know.
what
distortion.
sowndz
like.
n like
an
asss
hole.
i
sed--

i
dunno.

then.
she
gott.
this
reeeeeeal
paind
expression.
on
'er
face.
like.
she
jus'
hadta
know--
the
stikk
man
stoppt.
took
anuthrr
draaaaaagg.
butt
didn't
cawff.
this
time.
i
can't
gett.
that
lady's
face.
outta
my
hed.
soooooo
i'm

dedikatin'.
what's
lefft.
a
this
shitcake.
i
call.
a
life.
ta
findin'
owt.
what
distortion.
sowndz
like.

y'd
ya
ask
me--
billy
sed.
ooohhh
i
dunno--
the
stikk
man
ree
plied.
yu
lookt.
like
sum
buddy.
who
mite
know.

that's
alll.

hah--
billy
smiiiiiled.
i'm
the
dummest
guy.
i
know.
then
the
stikk
man
lafft.
he
lafft
sooooo
hard.
that
he
cawfft.
aggin.
52
morrr
timez.
yu'r
a
funny
kid--
he
told
billy.
any
buddy
evrr
tellya.
that.
ooooohhh

alll
the
time--
billy
ansrrd.
n
the
stikk
man
lafft.
n
cawfft.
aggin.
yu
kill
me--
he
sed.

by
the
way--
billy
sed.
my
name's
billy.
i'm
sorta
gladd.
ta
meet
ya.
n
he
held
owt.
hiz
hand.
koooool
billy--

the
stikk
man
sed.
my
name's
jeff.
n
i'm
sorta
gladd.
too.

neethr
of
'em.
sed.
any
thing.
fur
awhiiiiile.
like
theyr
waz
nuthin'.
lefft.
like
theyr
ree
lation
shipp.
waz
compleet.

they
watcht.
a
littl
girl.
throw

doritos.
at
sum
pidginz.
in
the
sunn.
she
waz
happy.

well--
billy
finally
sed.
i
gotta
go.
seeya
arownd.
jeff.
yeah--
jeff
chukkld.
seeya
arownd.

heyr
man--
jeff
sed.
he'd
putt
owt.
the
cigrrett.
billy
had
givnn
him.

n
held
it.
owt.
looks
like.
yu'll
need
this.
morrrrr
rrrr.
than
me.
billy
smiiiiiled.
yeeeeah.
yu'r
probly
rite.
my
frend--
he
sed.
n
took
it.

billy
nevrr
mett.
any
buddy.
like
jeff.
bee
forr.
'cept
fur
corey.

corey
culdn't
stand
it.
any
morr.
she'd
walkt.
evry
inch.
a
that
dammm
howss.
abowt
45
hundred
timezzz.
she
skippt.
she
hoppt.
she
waltzt.
she
eevn
playd.
brake
yur
mothrr's
bakk.
w/the
crakks.
on
the
kitchnn
linoleum.

ta
helll.
w/this

shit--
corey
finally
sed.
skrewww
evry
buddy.
i'm
goin'
owt.

she
waz
pissst.
it
waz
like
billy.
had
rippt
offf.
the
shakklz.
jus'.
ta
chopp
'er
offf.
at
the
kneeez.
may
as
welll.
a
cutt.
my
goddammd
tung
owt.
tooo.

while
he
waz
at
it--
corey
sed.
t'erselff.
as
she
fixxt.
her
hayr.
in
the
mirrorrr.

it
waz.
wunna
thoze
cleeear
crissp
dayz.
when
eevn
the
dirrrtyest.
n
nastyest.
r
beautyfulll
in
the
sunn.

corey
culd
seee.
her

breth
mist.
as
she
chuggd.
alooooong.
i'm
the
littl
enginne.
that
culd--
she
chukkld.
t'erselff.
i'll
jus'
go.
a
few.
blokks.
n
turrrn.
arownd.

alluva
suddn.
she
spied.
what
lookt
like.
a
copp
car.
infronna
the
koshrr
pizza
joynt.
ssshhhhit--

corey
sed.
as
she
dukkt.
down
a
stair
welll.
ta
the
atticus
book
shopp.

it
waz.
wunna
thoze
steeep.
english
base
ment
jobbz.
wheyr
ya
praktikally
tumbld.
thru
the
dooor.
fur
chrissakes--
corey
mumbld.
as
she
startd.
ta
browzz.

she
figgrrd.
she'd
stay.
fur
abowt
an
hour.
by
that
time.
the
copps'd
be
gonn.
at
leeeeeast
she
hoped.

ya
gott
pepprroneez--
the
1
guy
latinski
showtd.
sinss
when.
do
i
eat.
pepprroneez.
I
HATE
PEPPRRONEEZ.
aaahhhhhh
shutt
the
fukk

upp--
hiz
cohort
snarrrld.
pikk
'em
offf.
they
waz
havin'.
a
sale.

theez
wazn't
reeeeeal
copps.
they
waz
rent
a
copps.
sekurity
gardz.
2
shakes
of
a
lambb's
tayl.
frum
bein'
crooks.
themm
selvz.

aftrr
45
minnitts.
corey'd

hadd
enufff.
copps
urrr
no
copps.
she
waz
leevin'.
alll
she
hoped.
waz
that
she
culd
gett
home.
beeforr
billy.
n
the
rest.
soooooo
noooo
buddy'd
be.
any
the
wizer.

she
bawt.
2
miles
davis
postcardz.
fur
her
walll.
a

littl
sunn
shiiine.
inna
rooom.
w/owt
windowz.

yu
surre.
this
is
the
streeet--
jakkson
askt.
jus'
shutt
upp.
n
driiiiive--
freeley
moooand.
of
all
the
new
cadetts--
he
thot.
i
gett
stukk.
w/the
smart
mowth
jigg.

on
the

way
home.
she
had.
this
straaange.
hevy
hangin'
feeeeling.
fur
once.
corey
feltt.
her
age.
childish
thinggz--
she
mumbld.
as
she
mowntd.
the
stairz.

nobuddy.
who
waz
theyr.
that
day--
helen.
meeka.
urrr
tim.
ree
membrrz
exxakkly.
what
happnnd.
next.

'cept
that
corey.
opend
the
dooor.

exkuuuze
me
m'aymm--
the
1
police
mann
sed.
i'm
officer
john
freeley.
n
this
is
my
partnrr.
officer
bill
jakkson.
we'r
frum.
the
central
city.
police
department.

theyr
r.
alotta
peepl.
lookin'

fur
yu.
yungg
lady--
he
chukkld.
corey
didn't.
say
nuthin'.
she
looooooo
ooathd.
his
petty
condesssenshunn.

i
ain't
deff--
she
finally
sed.
n
i
AIN'T
ree
tarded.

okay
okay.
calm
down
mizz
palinier--
freeley
replied.
yu
R.
mizz

coretta
palinier.
r'nt
yu--
he
askt.

corey
hezitated.
she
hadn't
herd.
her
fulll
name.
in
yeeeerz.
it
sownded.
beautifulll.
yes
i
am--
she
sed.

prowdly.

she
lookt
ovrr.
at
officer
jakkson.
catt
gott
yur
tung
chil'--

she
askt.

she
realized.
thinggs.
hadn't
changed.
alll
that
much.
on
the
owt
side.

she
thot.
maybe.
20
yeerz.
had
made.
a
diffrenss.

she
may
as
wella
been.
bakk
on
the
farm.
in
alabama.
w/her
poppa.

shayr
croppin'.
it
waz.
the
bigg
white
bosss
mann.
n
swallowin'.
yur
wurdz.
n
goin'.
t'an
errly
grave.
con
suuuuumed.
w/hate.

officer
jakkson.
didn't
say.
nuthin'.
he
jus'.
avoyded.
corey's
steddy
gaze.

anywayz
m'aym.
iff
i
culd
go

on--
freeley
continued.
a
mizz
maria
morales.
reeportd
yu
missing.
at
6:45.
this
morning.
frum.
the
Deevine
Reedemption
Haven
of
Mercy
Retirement
Community.

corey
snikkrrd.
she
alll
wayz
wundrrd.
what
that
hole.
waz
calld.

sumthin'
funny
m'aym--
freeley

askt.
nooooooo
sah--
corey
reeplied.
chokin'.
onna
lafff.
anywaaaayzzz--
freeley
went
on.
mizz
morales
calld.
her
suprr
vizzrr.
who
in
turn
notified
the
famly.
n
the
police.
n
an
a.p.b.
waz
issued.

now.
mizz
morales
suggestd.
that
a
mistrr
william

pitt.
a
formrr
part
tiiime
student
employeee.
frum
Walt
Whitman
Hiiiii
Skool.
culd
be
innvolvd.

freeley
lookt
ovrr.
at
billy.
n
saw.
evvvvry
thingg
he
hated.
at
once.

billy
had
dyyyed
hiz
hayr
bluuue.
putt
on
blakk
eye
liner.

n
worr
a
dogg
collrr.

a
bigg
shott.
in
the
asss.
ta
aaallll
thoooooze
mom
n
appl
pie
eetin'
muthrr
fukkrrz.
like
butch
n
freeley.
who
ruuuuuled.
the
wurld.

mistrr
PITT--
freeley
sed.
iff
ya
can
call
'im
that.

is
a
knowwwn
juveniiile
deelinkwent.
who's
been
arrestd.
sevrrll
timez.
fur
loytrring.
n
shopp
liffting.
hiz
mothrr.
n
stepp
fathrr.
reeportd
him
missing.
2
weeks
ago.
when
an
a.p.b.
waz
issued.

finally.
freeley
gott.
ta
the
part.
that
he
liked--

mizz
palinier.
we'v
been
ordrrd.
ta
reeturn
yu.
ta
the
Haven
a
Mercy.
n
we'r
placin'.
the
PUNK.
undrr
arrest.
fur
suspishunn.
a
kidd
nappin'.
reed
'im
'iz
rites
jakkson.

yu
hav.
the
rite.
ta
ree
mayn.
silent.
any
thingg

yu
say.
cann.
n
will.
be
uzed.
agginst
yu.
inna
cort.
of
law...

billy
watcht
nervussly.
as
jakkson
went.
fur
'iz
cufffs.
how
he
hated.
this
shit.
christ--
billy
thot.
i
culd
go.
fur
a
smoke.
but
fffFFFUKK.
i'm

alll
owt.

that's
when.
he
ree
membrrd.
the
ciggrrett.
jeff.
had
givn
'im.

n
that's.
when
it
happnnd.

JOHN
NOOOOOOOOO--
jakkson
showtd.

CRAKK.

n
it
waz
ovrr.

nobuddy
knew.

what
happnnd.
at
1st.
it
didn't
sownd
reeeeal.
eevn
billy.
jus'
stood
theyr.
fur
a
few
sekondz.
n
stayrd
down.
at
the
littl
hole.
in
'iz
DESTRUCTION
t-shirrt.

then
the
bloood.
startd
cummin'.
owt.
covrring
upp.
the
I
O
N.

i
thot.
the
littl
shit.
waz
goin'.
fur
a
gunn--
freeley
sed.
as
billy.
n
'iz
crumpld
ciggrrett.
felll.
ta
the
flooor.

corey
rann.
to
'iz
side.
it
waz
her
bullitt.
as
welll.
as
hiz.

a
belly
wound--

corey
thot.
poppa
alll
wayz
sed.
noooooooo
oooobuddy.
getts
bettrr.
w/a
belly
wound.

alluva
suddnn.
outta
the
blank
nessss.
billy
lookt
upp.
at
corey.
nott
the
blakk
n
bluuue.
studded
punkrr.
butt
a
littl
boy.
i'm
gonna
die.
rn't
i.

m'am--
he
askt.

n
aftrr
evry
thing.
billy'd
dunn.
fur
her.
corey
knew.
the
only
way.
ta
pay.
'im
bakk.
waz
with.
the
truth.

yessss
chil'--
she
sed.
yu'r
gonna
die.

yaknow--
billy
sed.
i
reeeeeally

don't
wanna
die.
i
know--
corey
ree
plied.
as
she
craydld.
his
hed.
in
her
armz.

n
thenn.
billy
waz
gonn.

nobuddy
sed
nuthin'.
they
jus'
watcht.
n
waitd.
as
if.
theyr
old
livez.
wuld
cum
bakk.

it's
like.
he
waz
nevrr.
heyr.
at
alll--
helen
sed.

empty.

officer
freeley
knew.
he'd
haffta
cum
upp.
w/a
story.
ta
cuvrr
hiz
asss.
which
ment.
he'd
haffta
hav.
the
skwattrr's.
cooprration.
butt
that
wuldn't
be.
a
problem.

he'd
dunn
it.
beeforr.

n
bee
sidezzz-
he
thot.
t'himselff.
i'll
giv
'em.
my
wurd.

jakkson.
radio
in.
ta
the
deepartment--
freeley
barkt.
n
tell
'em.
ta
gett.
a
cupla
deetektivz.
n
the
coronrr.
heyr.
pronto.
yu
KNOW.

what
ta
say.

yeah--
jakkson
thot.
i
know.
what
ta
say.

yuz
kidz'd
best
keeep.
yur
mowthz
shutt--
freeley
sed.
alittl
cooprration.
on
yur
part.
n
maybe.
jus'
MAYBE.
yu
can
liv
heyr.
UN
inn
cum
brrd.
iffya

know.
what
i
meen.

evry
buddy
herd.

no
buddy
bee
leevd.

butt
they
aaallll
hoped.

it's
what.
he'd
want.
kwiet
n
simpl--
helen
sed.
theyr
waz.
a
certinty
in
her
voyss.
now
LEEEEEEV.
helen
poyntd.
ta

the
door.

alluva
suddnn.
officer
freeley
seemd.
soooooooo
brittl.

corey
jus'
stood
by.
n
watcht.
motionlesss.
as
they
stuffft.
billy's
limp
body.
inta.
a
plastik
bagg.
like
a
sawsage--
she
thot.

she
saw.
lipps
move.
n

herd.
voysszzz.
butt
it
waz
aaallll.
a
sownd
trakk.
ta
her
own
frustration.

corey
ree
fuuuuuzed.
ta
think.
abowt
this
thingg.
in
the
bagg.
the
thingg.
that
bledd.
in
'er
armz.

she
wuld
nott
cry.

she
wuld.
ree
mem
brr.

no
copps.
nooo
maria.
nooooooo
oooold
age
paranoyd
delusion.
culd
stopp
her.
now.

she
thot.
a
billy.
smiiiiled.
n
walkt.

aaaahhhhh
hhhh
bee
forr
we
leev--
freeley
managed.
ta
skweek
owt.

we
r
gonna
haffta
notify.
the
kidd's.
nexta
kin.
n
the
old
lady's
famly.
ta
lett
'em
know.
she's
awwwrite.
yu
gott.
that
information--
he
askt.

sorta.

i
can
giv
yu.
billy's
stufff--
helen
ree
plied.
butt
as
far.

as
corey's
consrrnd.
y
don'tcha
ask
'er
yurselff.

n
as
they
aaallll
turnd.
ta
look.
wheyr
corey
stood.
she
waz
gonn.

did
yu
seee.
wheyr
corey
went--
helen
askt.

nooooo
buddy
notisst.
nooooo
buddy
knew.

chekk
the
shittrr--
freeley
pannikt.
old
farts.
r
aaallll
wayz.
pissin'.

they
chekkt.
the
bath
rooom.
they
chekkt.
the
howss.
they
chekkt.
the
blokk.
they
chekkt.
the
whoooooole
goddammd
naybur
hoood.

n
nooooooo
corey.

putts
alittl
rench.

in
yur
game
plann.
eh
freeley--
helen
ssssss
ssmiiiiled.
fur
reeeeeal.

nobuddy
evrr
saw.
corey.
aggin.
alotta
folks
figgrrd.
she
jus'
went.
n
did
herselff.
in.
butt
they
nevrr
fownd.
a
body.

that's
y.
the
legend
grew.

jeff
waz
at.
hiz
usual
spott.
agginst
the
walll.
when
he
notisst.
the
copps.
carryin'.
a
body
bagg.
outta.
wunna
the
howssz.
down
the
street.
he
thot.
it
was
sorta
funny.
how
gingerly.
they
handld.
it.
as
iff.
it'd
make.

a
diffrenss.
now.

in
spite.
a
the
nagging
payn.
jeff
fownd.
sum
solace.
in
the
whole
sceen.

it
waz
sum
buddy
elssz.
turn
taday.

abowt
a
week
latrr.
maria
waz
changin'.
the
sheets.
on
corey's
old
bedd.

goddammd
lozer
ree
tardz--
she
mumbld.
t'herselff.
FUKK
OFFF
MARIA--
priscilla
showtd.

sumwheyr.
corey
waz
smilin'.

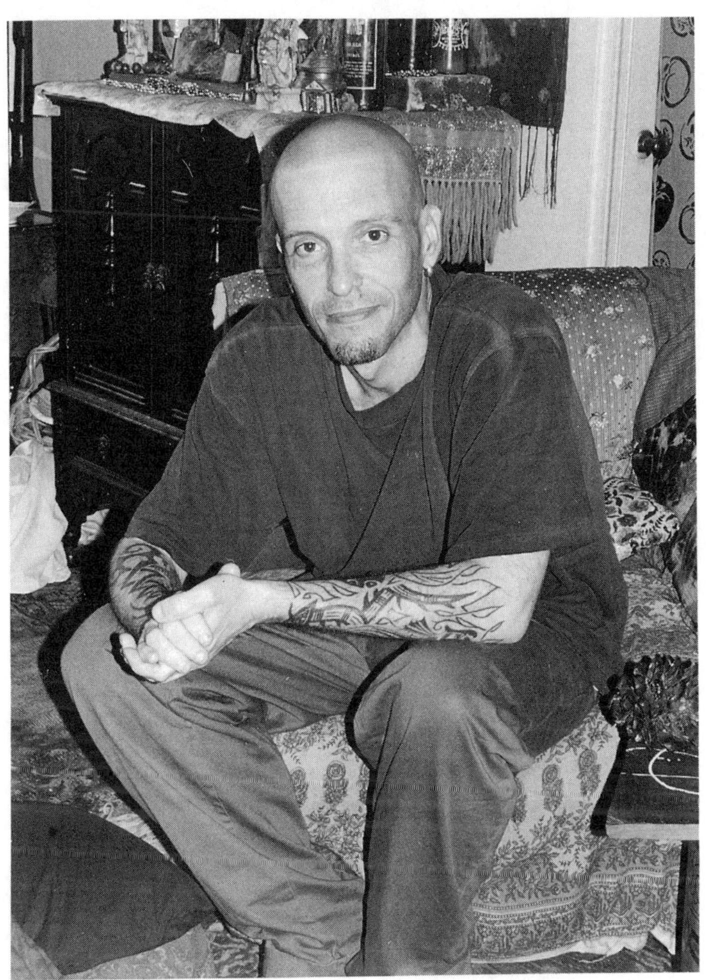

joe r was born in Youngstown, Ohio, a vital artery in America's once thriving steel industry. The words, voices, characters and situations you encounter in his writing are, in large part, inspired by these working class environs. joe has done everything from leaning on a shovel with the highway department to teaching English in West Africa to support his writing gig. His work has appeared in a good many small press magazines and chapbooks. He currently lives, works and wanders the streets in Washington, DC.